STAGE 4 RENAL DIET COOKBOOK FOR SENIORS

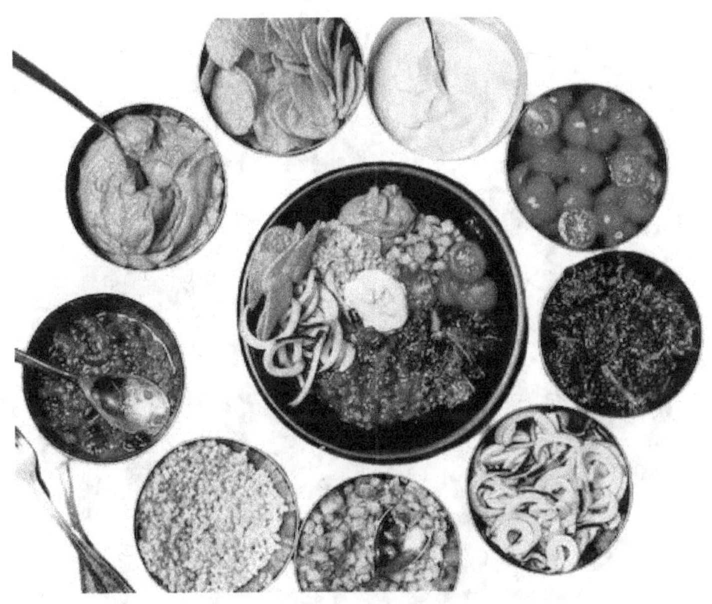

DR. VICKIE STOCK

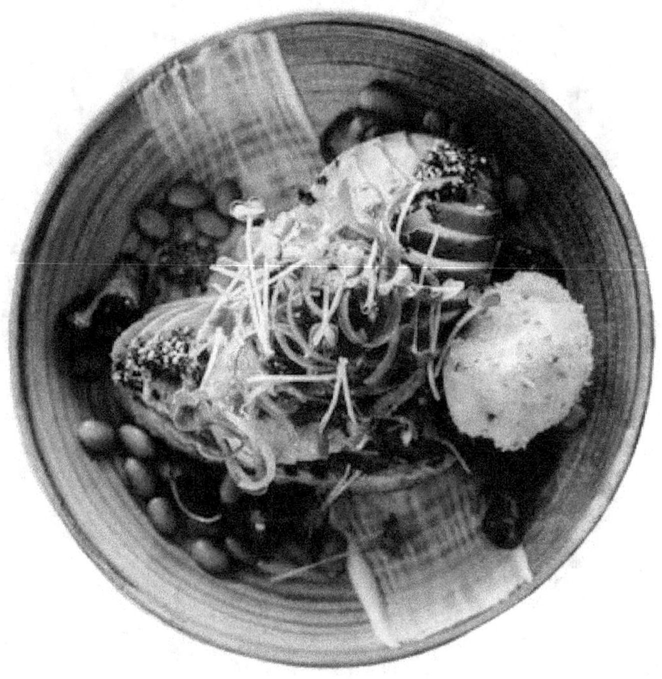

TABLE OF CONTENT

INTRODUCTION

Understanding Stage 4 CKD

Stage 4 Chronic Kidney Disease (CKD) represents a significant advancement in kidney dysfunction, characterized by severe impairment in kidney function. Understanding Stage 4 CKD is crucial for individuals and caregivers to effectively manage the condition and maintain quality of life.

At Stage 4 CKD, kidney function is notably reduced, with a glomerular filtration rate (GFR) ranging from 15 to 29 milliliters per minute per 1.73 square meters.

This stage signifies a critical point in the progression of kidney disease, where intervention and management become increasingly vital to prevent further deterioration and complications.

Symptoms and manifestations of Stage 4 CKD can vary among individuals but commonly include fatigue, swelling (edema), changes in urination patterns, decreased appetite, nausea, and difficulty concentrating.

Complications associated with Stage 4 CKD are numerous and can include hypertension, anemia, bone disease, cardiovascular disease, electrolyte imbalances, and fluid retention.

Regular monitoring of kidney function through blood tests, urine tests, and imaging studies is essential during Stage 4 CKD to track progression and guide treatment decisions. Additionally, lifestyle modifications such as dietary changes, fluid management, and medication adherence are key components of managing Stage 4 CKD.

Individuals with Stage 4 CKD often require close collaboration with healthcare professionals, including nephrologists, dietitians, and other specialists, to develop a comprehensive care plan tailored to their specific needs and circumstances.

Education about the condition, its progression, and strategies for slowing disease progression are essential for empowering individuals with CKD to actively participate in their care and improve outcomes.

CHAPTER ONE

Importance of Diet in Managing CKD

Diet plays a crucial role in managing Chronic Kidney Disease (CKD), especially in its advanced stages like Stage 4. A carefully planned diet can help slow the progression of CKD, alleviate symptoms, and reduce the risk of complications, ultimately improving the quality of life for individuals with CKD.

For individuals with Stage 4 CKD, dietary considerations are particularly important due to the significant decline in kidney function. The goals of a CKD-friendly diet at this stage typically include managing blood pressure, reducing the buildup of waste products and toxins in the blood, controlling fluid and electrolyte balance, and preserving overall nutritional status.

A key aspect of the CKD diet is controlling the intake of protein, phosphorus, potassium, sodium, and fluids. Protein intake may need to be restricted to reduce the workload on the kidneys, while phosphorus and potassium levels are often regulated to prevent imbalances that can lead to complications such as bone disease and cardiovascular issues.

Sodium restriction helps manage blood pressure and fluid retention, while fluid intake is often limited to prevent excessive fluid buildup in the body.

Additionally, individuals with Stage 4 CKD may benefit from monitoring their intake of other nutrients, such as calcium, vitamin D, and carbohydrates, to support overall health and well-being.

Working closely with a registered dietitian or nutritionist who specializes in kidney health is essential for developing a personalized CKD diet plan tailored to individual needs, preferences, and medical history.

With proper dietary management, individuals with Stage 4 CKD can optimize their nutritional intake, minimize symptoms, and improve their overall health outcomes.

How This Cookbook Can Help

This cookbook serves as a valuable resource for individuals navigating Stage 4 Chronic Kidney Disease (CKD) by providing a collection of renal-friendly recipes tailored specifically for seniors. Designed with their unique dietary needs and preferences in mind, this cookbook offers practical guidance and delicious meal options to support their overall health and well-being.

For seniors with Stage 4 CKD, adhering to a specialized diet is crucial for managing symptoms, preventing complications, and preserving kidney function. However, following dietary restrictions can often be challenging, especially when it comes to meal planning and preparation.

This cookbook aims to alleviate the stress and uncertainty associated with cooking for CKD by offering a diverse range of appetizing recipes that are not only kidney-friendly but also enjoyable and satisfying.

Each recipe included in this cookbook is carefully crafted to adhere to the dietary guidelines recommended for individuals with Stage 4 CKD. Ingredients are selected based on their nutritional value and their ability to support kidney health, while cooking methods are tailored to minimize the intake of substances that may exacerbate CKD symptoms.

By providing clear instructions, helpful tips, and nutritional information for each recipe, this cookbook empowers seniors with the knowledge and skills they need to make informed choices about their diet.

Whether they are seeking quick and easy meal ideas, looking to add variety to their diet, or simply wanting to enjoy flavorful dishes while managing their CKD, this cookbook offers a wealth of options to suit their tastes and preferences.

Ultimately, this cookbook aims to simplify the process of following a renal-friendly diet for seniors with Stage 4 CKD, enabling them to enjoy delicious and nourishing meals that support their health and well-being.

Stage 4 chronic kidney disease (CKD) is characterized by significant impairment in kidney function, typically with a glomerular filtration rate (GFR) of 15-29 mL/min/$1.73m^2$. The symptoms and complications associated with this stage can significantly impact a person's quality of life and require careful management.

One of the primary symptoms of Stage 4 CKD is fatigue. As kidney function declines, the body becomes less efficient at removing waste products and excess fluid from the blood. This can lead to a buildup of toxins and waste in the body, causing fatigue and weakness.

Other common symptoms include fluid retention, swelling (edema), shortness of breath, and changes in urination patterns. Individuals may experience increased frequency or decreased frequency of urination, foamy urine, or blood in the urine.

Complications of Stage 4 CKD can be serious and include cardiovascular disease, high blood pressure (hypertension), anemia, bone disease, and electrolyte imbalances. Cardiovascular disease is a leading cause of death in individuals with CKD, as kidney dysfunction can lead to an imbalance of minerals and hormones that regulate blood pressure and heart function.

Anemia is another significant complication of Stage 4 CKD, resulting from decreased production of red blood cells by the kidneys. This can lead to symptoms such as fatigue, weakness, and shortness of breath.

Bone disease is also common in individuals with Stage 4 CKD, as the kidneys play a crucial role in maintaining bone health by regulating calcium and phosphorus levels. As kidney function declines, bone mineral density may decrease, leading to an increased risk of fractures and bone pain.

Overall, the symptoms and complications of Stage 4 CKD highlight the importance of early detection and comprehensive management to slow the progression of the disease and improve quality of life.

Understanding Kidney Function

Understanding kidney function is crucial for managing chronic kidney disease (CKD), particularly in Stage 4, where significant impairment occurs. The kidneys play several vital roles in maintaining overall health and well-being.

Filtration: The primary function of the kidneys is to filter waste products and excess fluid from the blood to form urine. This process occurs in tiny structures called nephrons, which are the functional units of the kidneys. In Stage 4 CKD, the kidneys are functioning at a significantly reduced capacity, leading to a buildup of toxins and waste in the bloodstream.

Regulation of Fluid and Electrolytes: The kidneys help regulate the balance of fluids, electrolytes (such as sodium, potassium, and calcium), and acids in the body. In Stage 4 CKD, impaired kidney function can disrupt these balances, leading to fluid retention, electrolyte imbalances, and metabolic acidosis.

Blood Pressure Regulation: The kidneys play a crucial role in regulating blood pressure by controlling the amount of fluid in the bloodstream and releasing hormones that help narrow or widen blood vessels. In Stage 4 CKD, blood pressure may become difficult to control due to impaired kidney function, leading to hypertension and an increased risk of cardiovascular complications.

Production of Hormones: The kidneys produce several hormones that help regulate various bodily functions, including erythropoietin (EPO), which stimulates the production of red blood cells in the bone marrow. In Stage 4 CKD, the kidneys may produce insufficient amounts of EPO, leading to anemia.

Vitamin D Activation: The kidneys are responsible for converting vitamin D into its active form, which is essential for maintaining bone health and regulating calcium levels in the blood. In Stage 4 CKD, impaired kidney function can lead to vitamin D deficiency and bone disease.

CHAPTER TWO

Stage 4 Renal Diet Recipes for Seniors

BREAKFAST RECIPES:

1: Vegetable Omelette

Ingredients:

- 2 eggs
- 1/4 cup diced bell peppers
- 1/4 cup diced onions
- 1/4 cup diced tomatoes
- 1/4 cup chopped spinach
- Salt and pepper to taste
- 1 teaspoon olive oil

Instructions:

- In a bowl, beat the eggs and season with salt and pepper.
- Heat olive oil in a non-stick skillet over medium heat.
- Add bell peppers, onions, and tomatoes to the skillet and cook until softened.
- Add chopped spinach to the skillet and cook until wilted.
- Pour the beaten eggs over the vegetables in the skillet.

- Cook until the edges of the omelette start to set, then gently lift the edges and tilt the skillet to let the uncooked egg mixture flow underneath.
- Once the omelette is set, fold it in half and cook for another minute or until cooked through.
- Serve hot with a side of whole grain toast or a slice of low-sodium bread.

Health Benefits:

- High in protein from eggs, which is essential for muscle health.
- Packed with vitamins and minerals from vegetables, such as vitamin C, vitamin A, and folate.
- Low in sodium, potassium, and phosphorus, suitable for a renal diet.

Nutritional Value (per serving):

- Calories: 180 kcal
- Protein: 12g
- Carbohydrates: 7g
- Fat: 12g
- Fiber: 2g

Preparation Time: 15 minutes

2: Greek Yogurt Parfait

Ingredients:

- 1/2 cup plain Greek yogurt
- 1/4 cup fresh berries (such as strawberries, blueberries, or raspberries)
- 2 tablespoons chopped nuts (such as almonds or walnuts)
- 1 tablespoon honey (optional)

Instructions:

- In a glass or bowl, layer the Greek yogurt, fresh berries, and chopped nuts.
- Drizzle honey on top if desired for added sweetness.
- Repeat the layers if using a larger serving dish.
- Serve immediately or refrigerate until ready to eat.

Health Benefits:

- Greek yogurt is high in protein and calcium, which supports bone health.
- Berries are rich in antioxidants and fiber, promoting heart health and aiding digestion.
- Nuts provide healthy fats and additional protein, helping to keep you feeling full.

Nutritional Value (per serving):

- Calories: 200 kcal
- Protein: 12g
- Carbohydrates: 20g
- Fat: 8g
- Fiber: 4g

Preparation Time: 5 minutes

3: Avocado and Tomato Toast

Ingredients:

- 1 slice of whole grain bread
- 1/4 ripe avocado, mashed
- 1/4 cup diced tomatoes
- 1 teaspoon lemon juice
- Salt and pepper to taste
- 1 teaspoon olive oil (optional)

Instructions:

- Toast the whole grain bread until golden brown.
- In a small bowl, mix the mashed avocado with lemon juice, salt, and pepper.
- Spread the avocado mixture evenly on the toasted bread slice.

- Top with diced tomatoes and drizzle with olive oil if desired.
- Serve immediately.

Health Benefits:

- Whole grain bread provides fiber, which aids digestion and helps control blood sugar levels.
- Avocado is rich in heart-healthy monounsaturated fats and potassium.
- Tomatoes are a good source of vitamin C and antioxidants.

Nutritional Value (per serving):

- Calories: 150 kcal
- Protein: 4g
- Carbohydrates: 15g
- Fat: 9g
- Fiber: 5g

Preparation Time: 10 minutes

4: Spinach and Mushroom Frittata

Ingredients:

- 2 eggs
- 1/4 cup chopped spinach
- 1/4 cup sliced mushrooms
- 1 tablespoon diced onions

- 1 tablespoon grated Parmesan cheese
- Salt and pepper to taste
- 1 teaspoon olive oil

Instructions:

- Preheat the oven to 350°F (175°C).
- Heat olive oil in a non-stick skillet over medium heat.
- Add chopped spinach, sliced mushrooms, and diced onions to the skillet. Cook until vegetables are softened.
- In a bowl, beat the eggs and season with salt and pepper.
- Pour the beaten eggs over the cooked vegetables in the skillet.
- Sprinkle grated Parmesan cheese on top.
- Transfer the skillet to the preheated oven and bake for 10-12 minutes or until the frittata is set.
- Remove from the oven and let it cool for a few minutes before slicing.
- Serve warm.

Health Benefits:

- Eggs provide high-quality protein and essential nutrients like vitamin D and choline.
- Spinach is rich in iron and antioxidants, supporting overall health.

- Mushrooms are low in calories and a good source of B vitamins and minerals.

Nutritional Value (per serving):

- Calories: 180 kcal
- Protein: 12g
- Carbohydrates: 5g
- Fat: 12g
- Fiber: 2g

Preparation Time: 20 minutes

5: Greek Yogurt Parfait

Ingredients:

- 1/2 cup Greek yogurt (low-fat or non-fat)
- 1/4 cup mixed berries (such as blueberries, strawberries, raspberries)
- 1 tablespoon chopped walnuts or almonds
- 1 teaspoon honey (optional)
- 1 teaspoon ground flaxseed (optional)

Instructions:

- In a serving glass or bowl, layer Greek yogurt, mixed berries, and chopped nuts.
- Drizzle honey over the top if desired.

- Sprinkle ground flaxseed for added fiber and omega-3 fatty acids.

- Repeat the layers if using a larger serving dish.

- Serve chilled.

Health Benefits:

- Greek yogurt is high in protein and calcium, supporting bone health.

- Berries are rich in antioxidants and vitamins, promoting heart health and immunity.

- Nuts provide healthy fats and may help reduce inflammation.

Nutritional Value (per serving):

- Calories: 200 kcal

- Protein: 15g

- Carbohydrates: 20g

- Fat: 8g

- Fiber: 5g

Preparation Time: 5 minutes

6: Veggie Omelette

Ingredients:

- 2 eggs

- 1/4 cup diced bell peppers (any color)
- 1/4 cup diced zucchini
- 1 tablespoon diced onions
- 1 tablespoon chopped fresh parsley
- Salt and pepper to taste
- 1 teaspoon olive oil

Instructions:

- Heat olive oil in a non-stick skillet over medium heat.
- Add diced bell peppers, zucchini, and onions to the skillet. Cook until vegetables are tender.
- In a bowl, beat the eggs and season with salt, pepper, and chopped parsley.
- Pour the beaten eggs over the cooked vegetables in the skillet.
- Allow the eggs to set for a few minutes, then gently lift the edges with a spatula to let the uncooked egg flow underneath.
- Once the omelette is mostly set, fold it in half and cook for another minute until fully cooked through.
- Slide the omelette onto a plate and serve hot.

Health Benefits:

- Eggs provide essential amino acids and vitamins D and B12.

- Bell peppers and zucchini are low in calories and high in vitamins and antioxidants.
- Parsley adds flavor and contains vitamin K and antioxidants.

Nutritional Value (per serving):

- Calories: 180 kcal
- Protein: 12g
- Carbohydrates: 6g
- Fat: 12g
- Fiber: 2g

Preparation Time: 15 minutes

7: Avocado and Tomato Toast

Ingredients:

- 1 slice whole-grain bread (low-sodium if available)
- 1/4 ripe avocado, mashed
- 1 small tomato, sliced
- 1 teaspoon balsamic glaze (optional)
- Fresh basil leaves, for garnish
- Salt and pepper to taste

Instructions:

- Toast the slice of whole-grain bread until lightly browned.
- Spread the mashed avocado evenly over the toast.

- Arrange the tomato slices on top of the avocado.

- Drizzle with balsamic glaze if using.

- Season with salt and pepper to taste.

- Garnish with fresh basil leaves.

- Serve immediately.

Health Benefits:

- Avocado provides heart-healthy monounsaturated fats and potassium.

- Tomatoes are rich in lycopene, an antioxidant associated with reduced risk of chronic diseases.

- Whole-grain bread offers fiber for digestive health and sustained energy.

Nutritional Value (per serving):

- Calories: 180 kcal

- Protein: 5g

- Carbohydrates: 20g

- Fat: 9g

- Fiber: 6g

Preparation Time: 10 minutes

8: Chia Seed Pudding

Ingredients:

- 2 tablespoons chia seeds
- 1/2 cup unsweetened almond milk (or any milk of choice)
- 1/4 teaspoon vanilla extract
- 1 teaspoon honey or maple syrup (optional)
- Fresh berries for topping (optional)

Instructions:

- In a bowl or jar, combine chia seeds, almond milk, vanilla extract, and sweetener if using.
- Stir well to mix all ingredients.
- Cover and refrigerate for at least 2 hours or overnight until the mixture thickens and forms a pudding-like consistency.
- Before serving, stir the chia pudding to redistribute the seeds.
- Top with fresh berries if desired.
- Serve chilled.

Health Benefits:

- Chia seeds are high in fiber, omega-3 fatty acids, and antioxidants.
- Almond milk is low in calories and contains vitamin E and calcium.

- Berries provide vitamins, minerals, and phytochemicals with various health benefits.

Nutritional Value (per serving):

- Calories: 120 kcal
- Protein: 4g
- Carbohydrates: 12g
- Fat: 7g
- Fiber: 8g

Preparation Time: 5 minutes (plus chilling time)

9: Greek Yogurt Parfait

Ingredients:

- 1/2 cup plain Greek yogurt
- 1/4 cup low-carb granola
- 1/4 cup mixed fresh berries (such as strawberries, blueberries, raspberries)
- 1 tablespoon chopped nuts (such as almonds or walnuts)
- 1 teaspoon honey or maple syrup (optional)

Instructions:

- In a serving glass or bowl, layer the Greek yogurt, granola, and mixed berries.

- Repeat the layers until ingredients are used up, ending with a layer of berries on top.
- Sprinkle chopped nuts over the berries.
- Drizzle honey or maple syrup over the parfait if desired.
- Serve immediately or refrigerate until ready to eat.

Health Benefits:

- Greek yogurt provides protein, calcium, and probiotics for gut health.
- Berries are rich in antioxidants and fiber, supporting heart and digestive health.
- Nuts offer healthy fats, protein, and micronutrients like vitamin E and magnesium.

Nutritional Value (per serving):

- Calories: 250 kcal
- Protein: 15g
- Carbohydrates: 25g
- Fat: 10g
- Fiber: 6g

Preparation Time: 5 minutes

10: Veggie Omelette

Ingredients:

- 2 large eggs
- 1/4 cup chopped mixed vegetables (bell peppers, onions, spinach, mushrooms)
- 1 tablespoon chopped fresh herbs (such as parsley or chives)
- 1 teaspoon olive oil
- Salt and pepper to taste
- 2 tablespoons shredded low-fat cheese (optional)

Instructions:

- In a bowl, beat the eggs with a fork until well mixed.
- Heat olive oil in a non-stick skillet over medium heat.
- Add the chopped vegetables and sauté until softened, about 2-3 minutes.
- Pour the beaten eggs into the skillet, tilting to spread evenly.
- Cook the omelette for 2-3 minutes, or until the edges start to set.
- Sprinkle chopped herbs, salt, pepper, and shredded cheese (if using) over one half of the omelette.
- Carefully fold the other half of the omelette over the filling.
- Cook for another 1-2 minutes until the cheese melts and the omelette is cooked through.

- Slide the omelette onto a plate and serve hot.

Health Benefits:

- Eggs provide high-quality protein and essential nutrients like choline and vitamin D.
- Mixed vegetables offer vitamins, minerals, and fiber for overall health and digestion.
- Olive oil provides heart-healthy monounsaturated fats and antioxidants.

Nutritional Value (per serving):

- Calories: 220 kcal
- Protein: 15g
- Carbohydrates: 5g
- Fat: 15g
- Fiber: 2g

Preparation Time: 10 minutes

LUNCH RECIPES:

1: Quinoa Salad with Chickpeas and Vegetables

Ingredients:

- 1/2 cup cooked quinoa
- 1/2 cup cooked chickpeas (canned, rinsed, and drained)
- 1/4 cup diced cucumber

- 1/4 cup diced bell peppers (any color)
- 1/4 cup halved cherry tomatoes
- 2 tablespoons chopped fresh parsley
- 1 tablespoon extra-virgin olive oil
- 1 tablespoon lemon juice
- Salt and pepper to taste

Instructions:

- In a large bowl, combine the cooked quinoa, chickpeas, cucumber, bell peppers, cherry tomatoes, and parsley.
- Drizzle the olive oil and lemon juice over the salad.
- Season with salt and pepper to taste.
- Toss everything together until well combined.
- Serve immediately or refrigerate until ready to eat.

Health Benefits:

- Quinoa is a good source of plant-based protein and fiber.
- Chickpeas provide protein, fiber, and essential nutrients like folate and iron.
- Vegetables offer vitamins, minerals, and antioxidants for overall health.

Nutritional Value (per serving):

- Calories: 250 kcal

- Protein: 10g

- Carbohydrates: 35g

- Fat: 8g

- Fiber: 8g

Preparation Time: 15 minutes

2: Mediterranean Vegetable Wrap

Ingredients:

- 1 whole wheat tortilla or wrap

- 1/4 cup hummus

- 1/4 cup mixed salad greens

- 1/4 cup sliced cucumber

- 1/4 cup sliced bell peppers (any color)

- 1/4 cup shredded carrots

- 2 tablespoons crumbled feta cheese (optional)

- 1 tablespoon chopped fresh herbs (such as parsley or dill)

Instructions:

- Spread the hummus evenly over the whole wheat tortilla.

- Layer the mixed salad greens, sliced cucumber, bell peppers, shredded carrots, crumbled feta cheese (if using), and chopped fresh herbs on top of the hummus.

- Roll up the tortilla tightly, tucking in the sides as you go.

- Cut the wrap in half diagonally before serving, if desired.
- Serve immediately or wrap in foil for later.

Health Benefits: Whole wheat tortilla provides complex carbohydrates and fiber.

- Hummus offers plant-based protein, fiber, and healthy fats.
- Vegetables contribute vitamins, minerals, and antioxidants.

Nutritional Value (per serving):

- Calories: 280 kcal
- Protein: 10g
- Carbohydrates: 35g
- Fat: 10g
- Fiber: 8g

Preparation Time: 10 minutes

3: Lentil and Vegetable Soup

Ingredients:

- 1/2 cup dried green lentils, rinsed and drained
- 4 cups low-sodium vegetable broth
- 1 cup diced carrots
- 1 cup diced celery
- 1 cup diced zucchini
- 1/2 cup diced onion

- 2 cloves garlic, minced

- 1 teaspoon dried thyme

- 1 teaspoon dried oregano

- Salt and pepper to taste

- Fresh parsley for garnish (optional)

Instructions:

- In a large pot, combine the vegetable broth, lentils, carrots, celery, zucchini, onion, garlic, thyme, and oregano.

- Bring the mixture to a boil over medium-high heat.

- Reduce the heat to low, cover, and simmer for about 20-25 minutes or until the lentils and vegetables are tender.

- Season with salt and pepper to taste.

- Serve hot, garnished with fresh parsley if desired.

Health Benefits:

- Lentils are rich in protein, fiber, and minerals like iron and folate.

- Vegetables provide vitamins, minerals, and antioxidants.

- This soup is low in sodium and cholesterol-free, making it heart-healthy.

Nutritional Value (per serving):

- Calories: 200 kcal

- Protein: 12g

- Carbohydrates: 35g

- Fat: 1g

- Fiber: 10g

Preparation Time: 30 minutes

4: Grilled Vegetable Salad with Balsamic Vinaigrette

Ingredients:

- 1 small eggplant, sliced into rounds

- 1 zucchini, sliced lengthwise

- 1 yellow squash, sliced lengthwise

- 1 red bell pepper, quartered

- 1 yellow bell pepper, quartered

- 1/4 cup balsamic vinegar

- 2 tablespoons extra-virgin olive oil

- 1 teaspoon Dijon mustard

- 1 clove garlic, minced

- Salt and pepper to taste

- Fresh basil leaves for garnish (optional)

Instructions:

- Preheat the grill to medium-high heat.

- In a small bowl, whisk together the balsamic vinegar, olive oil, Dijon mustard, minced garlic, salt, and pepper to make the vinaigrette.
- Brush the eggplant, zucchini, squash, and bell peppers with the vinaigrette.
- Grill the vegetables for 3-4 minutes on each side or until tender and lightly charred.
- Arrange the grilled vegetables on a serving platter.
- Drizzle with the remaining vinaigrette and garnish with fresh basil leaves if desired.
- Serve warm or at room temperature.

Health Benefits:

- Grilled vegetables are low in calories and fat but rich in vitamins, minerals, and antioxidants.
- Balsamic vinaigrette adds flavor without extra sodium.

Nutritional Value (per serving):

- Calories: 180 kcal
- Protein: 5g
- Carbohydrates: 20g
- Fat: 10g
- Fiber: 8g

Preparation Time: 20 minutes

5: Lentil and Vegetable Soup

Ingredients:

- 1/2 cup dried green lentils
- 4 cups low-sodium vegetable broth
- 1/2 cup diced carrots
- 1/2 cup diced celery
- 1/2 cup diced zucchini
- 1/2 cup diced onion
- 2 cloves garlic, minced
- 1 teaspoon dried thyme
- 1 teaspoon dried oregano
- Salt and pepper to taste
- 2 tablespoons chopped fresh parsley (for garnish)

Instructions:

- Rinse the lentils under cold water and drain.
- In a large pot, combine the lentils, vegetable broth, carrots, celery, zucchini, onion, garlic, thyme, and oregano.
- Bring the mixture to a boil over medium-high heat, then reduce the heat to low and simmer for about 20-25 minutes, or until the lentils and vegetables are tender.
- Season with salt and pepper to taste.

- Ladle the soup into bowls and garnish with chopped fresh parsley before serving.

Health Benefits:

- Lentils are a good source of plant-based protein, fiber, and essential nutrients like folate and iron.
- Vegetables add vitamins, minerals, and antioxidants to support kidney health.
- Low-sodium vegetable broth helps control blood pressure and fluid balance.

Nutritional Value (per serving):

- Calories: 200 kcal
- Protein: 12g
- Carbohydrates: 35g
- Fat: 1g
- Fiber: 12g

Preparation Time: 30 minutes

6: Greek Chickpea Salad

Ingredients:

- 1 can (15 ounces) chickpeas, rinsed and drained
- 1 cup diced cucumber
- 1 cup halved cherry tomatoes

- 1/4 cup diced red onion

- 1/4 cup chopped fresh parsley

- 2 tablespoons crumbled feta cheese (optional)

- 2 tablespoons extra-virgin olive oil

- 1 tablespoon lemon juice

- 1 teaspoon dried oregano

- Salt and pepper to taste

Instructions:

- In a large bowl, combine the chickpeas, cucumber, cherry tomatoes, red onion, parsley, and feta cheese (if using).

- Drizzle the olive oil and lemon juice over the salad.

- Sprinkle the dried oregano, salt, and pepper on top.

- Toss everything together until well combined.

- Serve immediately or refrigerate until ready to eat.

Health Benefits:

- Chickpeas provide protein, fiber, and essential nutrients.

- Vegetables offer vitamins, minerals, and antioxidants.

- Olive oil contributes heart-healthy fats and anti-inflammatory properties.

Nutritional Value (per serving):

- Calories: 220 kcal

- Protein: 8g

- Carbohydrates: 30g

- Fat: 8g

- Fiber: 8g

Preparation Time: 15 minutes

7: Eggplant and Tomato Stew

Ingredients:

- 1 large eggplant, diced

- 2 cups diced tomatoes (fresh or canned)

- 1 onion, chopped

- 2 cloves garlic, minced

- 1 tablespoon olive oil

- 1 teaspoon dried basil

- 1 teaspoon dried oregano

- Salt and pepper to taste

- Fresh basil leaves for garnish (optional)

Instructions:

- Heat olive oil in a large pot over medium heat. Add the chopped onion and minced garlic, sauté until softened.

- Add the diced eggplant to the pot and cook for about 5 minutes, stirring occasionally.

- Stir in the diced tomatoes, dried basil, dried oregano, salt, and pepper.

- Bring the mixture to a simmer, then reduce the heat to low and cover the pot. Let it cook for about 20-25 minutes, or until the eggplant is tender.

- Adjust seasoning if needed. Serve hot, garnished with fresh basil leaves if desired.

- Health Benefits:

- Eggplant is low in potassium and high in fiber, making it suitable for a renal diet.

- Tomatoes provide antioxidants like lycopene and vitamins C and K.

- Olive oil offers heart-healthy monounsaturated fats.

Nutritional Value (per serving):

- Calories: 120 kcal

- Protein: 2g

- Carbohydrates: 15g

- Fat: 6g

- Fiber: 6g

Preparation Time: 35 minutes

8: Quinoa and Black Bean Salad

Ingredients:

- 1 cup cooked quinoa

- 1 can (15 ounces) black beans, rinsed and drained

- 1 cup diced bell peppers (red, yellow, or orange)

1/2 cup chopped fresh cilantro

- 1/4 cup chopped green onions

- 1/4 cup diced avocado

- 2 tablespoons lime juice

- 1 tablespoon extra-virgin olive oil

- 1 teaspoon ground cumin

- Salt and pepper to taste

Instructions:

- In a large bowl, combine the cooked quinoa, black beans, diced bell peppers, chopped cilantro, green onions, and diced avocado.

- In a small bowl, whisk together the lime juice, olive oil, ground cumin, salt, and pepper to make the dressing.

- Pour the dressing over the quinoa mixture and toss until well combined.

- Serve immediately or refrigerate for about 30 minutes to allow the flavors to meld before serving.

Health Benefits:

- Quinoa is a complete protein and a good source of fiber.
- Black beans offer protein, fiber, and essential minerals like iron and magnesium.
- Bell peppers provide vitamin C and antioxidants.

Nutritional Value (per serving):

- Calories: 200 kcal
- Protein: 8g
- Carbohydrates: 30g
- Fat: 6g
- Fiber: 8g

Preparation Time: 25 minutes

9: Quinoa and Roasted Vegetable Salad

Ingredients:

- 1 cup quinoa, rinsed
- 2 cups water or low-sodium vegetable broth
- 1 cup diced bell peppers (assorted colors)
- 1 cup diced eggplant
- 1 cup diced zucchini
- 1 cup cherry tomatoes, halved
- 1/4 cup diced red onion

- 2 tablespoons chopped fresh basil
- 2 tablespoons balsamic vinegar
- 2 tablespoons extra-virgin olive oil
- Salt and pepper to taste

Instructions:

- Preheat the oven to 400°F (200°C). Line a baking sheet with parchment paper.
- In a medium saucepan, bring the water or vegetable broth to a boil. Add the quinoa, reduce the heat to low, cover, and simmer for 15-20 minutes, or until the quinoa is cooked and the liquid is absorbed.
- Meanwhile, spread the diced bell peppers, eggplant, and zucchini on the prepared baking sheet. Drizzle with olive oil and season with salt and pepper. Roast in the preheated oven for 20-25 minutes, or until the vegetables are tender and lightly browned.
- In a large bowl, combine the cooked quinoa, roasted vegetables, cherry tomatoes, red onion, and chopped basil.
- Drizzle the balsamic vinegar and olive oil over the salad. Toss gently to combine.
- Serve the salad warm or at room temperature.

Health Benefits: Quinoa is a complete protein source and provides essential amino acids.

- Roasted vegetables offer vitamins, minerals, and antioxidants.
- Olive oil and balsamic vinegar add heart-healthy fats and flavor.

Nutritional Value (per serving):

- Calories: 250 kcal
- Protein: 7g
- Carbohydrates: 35g
- Fat: 10g
- Fiber: 6g

Preparation Time: 40 minutes

10: Stuffed Bell Peppers

Ingredients:

- 4 large bell peppers (any color), halved and seeds removed
- 1 cup cooked quinoa
- 1 can (15 ounces) low-sodium black beans, rinsed and drained
- 1 cup diced tomatoes
- 1/2 cup diced red onion
- 1/2 cup chopped fresh cilantro
- 1 teaspoon ground cumin

- 1/2 teaspoon chili powder

- Salt and pepper to taste

- 1/2 cup shredded low-fat cheese (optional)

Instructions:

- Preheat the oven to 375°F (190°C). Arrange the halved bell peppers in a baking dish, cut side up.

- In a large bowl, combine the cooked quinoa, black beans, diced tomatoes, red onion, cilantro, ground cumin, chili powder, salt, and pepper.

- Spoon the quinoa mixture evenly into each bell pepper half.

- If using cheese, sprinkle it over the stuffed peppers.

- Cover the baking dish with aluminum foil and bake in the preheated oven for 25-30 minutes, or until the peppers are tender.

- Remove the foil and bake for an additional 5 minutes to melt the cheese (if using).

- Serve the stuffed bell peppers hot.

Health Benefits:

- Bell peppers are rich in vitamin C and antioxidants.

- Quinoa and black beans provide protein, fiber, and essential nutrients.

- This dish is low in carbohydrates and contains no added sugars.

Nutritional Value (per serving, 1 stuffed pepper half):

- Calories: 180 kcal
- Protein: 8g
- Carbohydrates: 30g
- Fat: 3g
- Fiber: 7g

Preparation Time: 45 minutes

DINNER RECIPES:

1: Baked Lemon Herb Salmon

Ingredients:

- 2 salmon fillets (about 4-6 ounces each)
- 2 tablespoons fresh lemon juice
- 1 tablespoon olive oil
- 2 cloves garlic, minced
- 1 teaspoon dried thyme
- 1 teaspoon dried rosemary
- Salt and pepper to taste
- Lemon slices for garnish
- Fresh parsley, chopped, for garnish

Instructions: Preheat the oven to 400°F (200°C). Line a baking sheet with parchment paper.

- In a small bowl, whisk together the lemon juice, olive oil, minced garlic, dried thyme, dried rosemary, salt, and pepper.
- Place the salmon fillets on the prepared baking sheet. Brush the lemon herb mixture evenly over the salmon.
- Bake in the preheated oven for 12-15 minutes, or until the salmon is cooked through and flakes easily with a fork.
- Remove from the oven and garnish with lemon slices and chopped parsley before serving.

Health Benefits:

- Salmon is rich in omega-3 fatty acids, which are beneficial for heart health and reducing inflammation.
- Lemon juice adds flavor and provides vitamin C, an antioxidant that supports immune function.
- Herbs like thyme and rosemary offer antioxidants and antimicrobial properties.

Nutritional Value (per serving):

- Calories: 300 kcal
- Protein: 25g
- Carbohydrates: 2g
- Fat: 20g

- Fiber: 0g

Preparation Time: 20 minutes

2: Mediterranean Chickpea Salad

Ingredients:

- 2 cups cooked chickpeas (canned or cooked from dry)
- 1 cup cherry tomatoes, halved
- 1 cucumber, diced
- 1/2 red onion, thinly sliced
- 1/4 cup chopped fresh parsley
- 2 tablespoons chopped fresh mint
- 1/4 cup crumbled feta cheese (optional)
- 2 tablespoons extra-virgin olive oil
- 1 tablespoon fresh lemon juice
- 1 teaspoon dried oregano
- Salt and pepper to taste

Instructions:

- In a large mixing bowl, combine the cooked chickpeas, cherry tomatoes, diced cucumber, sliced red onion, chopped parsley, and chopped mint.
- If using, add the crumbled feta cheese to the bowl.

- In a small bowl, whisk together the olive oil, lemon juice, dried oregano, salt, and pepper to make the dressing.
- Pour the dressing over the salad ingredients and toss gently to combine.
- Taste and adjust seasoning if necessary.
- Serve the Mediterranean chickpea salad chilled or at room temperature.

Health Benefits:

- Chickpeas are a good source of plant-based protein and fiber.
- Tomatoes provide vitamin C and antioxidants, while cucumbers offer hydration and vitamins.
- Olive oil contributes heart-healthy monounsaturated fats, and fresh herbs add flavor and nutrients.

Nutritional Value (per serving):

- Calories: 250 kcal
- Protein: 10g
- Carbohydrates: 30g
- Fat: 10g
- Fiber: 8g

Preparation Time: 15 minutes

3: Grilled Vegetable Quinoa Bowl

Ingredients:

- 1 cup quinoa, rinsed
- 2 cups vegetable broth
- 2 cups mixed vegetables (such as bell peppers, zucchini, eggplant, and mushrooms), sliced
- 2 tablespoons olive oil
- 2 cloves garlic, minced
- 1 teaspoon dried Italian herbs
- Salt and pepper to taste
- 1/4 cup crumbled goat cheese (optional)
- Fresh basil leaves for garnish

Instructions:

- In a medium saucepan, combine the quinoa and vegetable broth. Bring to a boil, then reduce heat to low, cover, and simmer for 15-20 minutes, or until the quinoa is tender and the liquid is absorbed.
- While the quinoa is cooking, preheat a grill pan or outdoor grill over medium-high heat.
- In a large bowl, toss the sliced mixed vegetables with olive oil, minced garlic, dried Italian herbs, salt, and pepper until evenly coated.

- Grill the vegetables for 5-7 minutes on each side, or until they are tender and have grill marks.
- To assemble the bowls, divide the cooked quinoa among serving bowls. Top with grilled vegetables and crumbled goat cheese, if using.
- Garnish with fresh basil leaves before serving.

Health Benefits:

- Quinoa provides a good source of protein and fiber.
- Grilled vegetables offer vitamins, minerals, and antioxidants.
- Olive oil contributes heart-healthy monounsaturated fats, and garlic adds flavor and potential health benefits.

Nutritional Value (per serving):

- Calories: 300 kcal
- Protein: 9g
- Carbohydrates: 40g
- Fat: 12g
- Fiber: 6g

Preparation Time: 30 minutes

4: Lentil and Vegetable Stew

Ingredients:

- 1 cup dried lentils, rinsed
- 4 cups vegetable broth
- 2 carrots, diced
- 2 celery stalks, diced
- 1 onion, diced
- 2 cloves garlic, minced
- 1 teaspoon dried thyme
- 1 teaspoon smoked paprika
- 1 bay leaf
- Salt and pepper to taste
- Fresh parsley, chopped, for garnish

Instructions:

- In a large pot, combine the dried lentils, vegetable broth, diced carrots, diced celery, diced onion, minced garlic, dried thyme, smoked paprika, bay leaf, salt, and pepper.
- Bring the mixture to a boil over medium-high heat. Reduce the heat to low, cover, and simmer for 25-30 minutes, or until the lentils and vegetables are tender.
- Remove the bay leaf from the stew before serving.

- Ladle the lentil and vegetable stew into bowls and garnish with chopped fresh parsley.

Health Benefits:

- Lentils are rich in plant-based protein and fiber.
- Carrots, celery, and onions provide vitamins, minerals, and antioxidants.
- Herbs and spices add flavor and potential health benefits.

Nutritional Value (per serving):

- Calories: 250 kcal
- Protein: 15g
- Carbohydrates: 45g
- Fat: 1g
- Fiber: 10g

Preparation Time: 40 minutes

5: Baked Salmon with Roasted Vegetables

Ingredients:

- 2 salmon fillets
- 1 small zucchini, sliced
- 1 small yellow squash, sliced
- 1 bell pepper, sliced
- 1 small red onion, sliced

- 2 tablespoons olive oil

- 2 cloves garlic, minced

- 1 teaspoon dried thyme

- Salt and pepper to taste

- Lemon wedges for serving

- Fresh parsley, chopped, for garnish

Instructions:

- Preheat the oven to 400°F (200°C). Line a baking sheet with parchment paper or aluminum foil.

- Arrange the salmon fillets and sliced vegetables on the prepared baking sheet.

- In a small bowl, whisk together the olive oil, minced garlic, dried thyme, salt, and pepper. Drizzle this mixture over the salmon and vegetables, ensuring they are evenly coated.

- Bake in the preheated oven for 15-20 minutes, or until the salmon is cooked through and the vegetables are tender.

- Remove from the oven and garnish with chopped parsley. Serve with lemon wedges on the side.

Health Benefits:

- Salmon is rich in omega-3 fatty acids, which have anti-inflammatory properties and support heart health.

- Vegetables like zucchini, squash, bell pepper, and onion provide vitamins, minerals, and fiber.
- Olive oil offers monounsaturated fats and antioxidants.

Nutritional Value (per serving):

- Calories: 300 kcal
- Protein: 25g
- Carbohydrates: 10g
- Fat: 18g
- Fiber: 4g

Preparation Time: 30 minutes

6: Quinoa Stuffed Bell Peppers

Ingredients:

- 4 large bell peppers, tops removed and seeds removed
- 1 cup cooked quinoa
- 1 can (15 ounces) black beans, drained and rinsed
- 1 cup diced tomatoes
- 1 cup diced zucchini
- 1/2 cup diced red onion
- 1/2 cup corn kernels (fresh or frozen)
- 1 teaspoon cumin
- 1 teaspoon chili powder

- Salt and pepper to taste

- 1/2 cup shredded cheddar cheese (optional)

- Fresh cilantro, chopped, for garnish

Instructions:

- Preheat the oven to 375°F (190°C). Grease a baking dish with olive oil or cooking spray.

- In a large bowl, mix together the cooked quinoa, black beans, diced tomatoes, diced zucchini, diced red onion, corn kernels, cumin, chili powder, salt, and pepper.

- Stuff each bell pepper with the quinoa and vegetable mixture, pressing down gently to pack it in.

- Place the stuffed bell peppers in the prepared baking dish. If using cheese, sprinkle it over the tops of the peppers.

- Cover the baking dish with foil and bake in the preheated oven for 30-35 minutes, or until the peppers are tender.

- Remove from the oven and garnish with chopped cilantro before serving.

Health Benefits:

- Quinoa is a complete protein, providing all nine essential amino acids.

- Black beans are high in fiber and protein, which can help regulate blood sugar levels.

- Bell peppers are rich in vitamin C and antioxidants.

Nutritional Value (per serving):

- Calories: 280 kcal
- Protein: 14g
- Carbohydrates: 45g
- Fat: 5g
- Fiber: 10g

Preparation Time: 45 minutes

7: Eggplant Parmesan

Ingredients:

- 1 large eggplant, sliced into rounds
- 1 cup whole wheat breadcrumbs
- 1/2 cup grated Parmesan cheese
- 2 eggs, beaten
- 2 cups marinara sauce
- 1 cup shredded mozzarella cheese
- 2 tablespoons olive oil
- Salt and pepper to taste
- Fresh basil leaves for garnish

Instructions: Preheat the oven to 375°F (190°C). Grease a baking sheet with olive oil or cooking spray.

- In a shallow dish, combine the whole wheat breadcrumbs and grated Parmesan cheese. Dip each eggplant slice into the beaten eggs, then coat it in the breadcrumb mixture.

- Place the coated eggplant slices on the prepared baking sheet. Drizzle with olive oil and season with salt and pepper.

- Bake in the preheated oven for 20-25 minutes, or until the eggplant is tender and golden brown.

- Remove the eggplant slices from the oven and top each with marinara sauce and shredded mozzarella cheese.

- Return the baking sheet to the oven and bake for an additional 10-15 minutes, or until the cheese is melted and bubbly.

- Garnish with fresh basil leaves before serving.

Health Benefits:

- Eggplant is low in calories and rich in fiber, vitamins, and minerals.

- Whole wheat breadcrumbs provide fiber and complex carbohydrates.

- Marinara sauce offers lycopene, a powerful antioxidant.

Nutritional Value (per serving):

- Calories: 250 kcal

- Protein: 12g

- Carbohydrates: 25g

- Fat: 12g

- Fiber: 6g

Preparation Time: 45 minutes

8: Lentil Vegetable Soup

Ingredients:

- 1 cup dry green lentils, rinsed and drained

- 4 cups vegetable broth

- 1 onion, diced

- 2 carrots, diced

- 2 celery stalks, diced

- 2 cloves garlic, minced

- 1 can (14 ounces) diced tomatoes

- 2 cups chopped spinach

- 1 teaspoon dried thyme

- 1 teaspoon dried oregano

- Salt and pepper to taste

- Fresh parsley, chopped, for garnish

Instructions:

- In a large pot, combine the vegetable broth, diced onion, diced carrots, diced celery, minced garlic, diced tomatoes, dried thyme, and dried oregano. Bring to a boil over medium-high heat.

- Reduce the heat to low and add the rinsed green lentils to the pot. Simmer for 20-25 minutes, or until the lentils and vegetables are tender.
- Stir in the chopped spinach and cook for an additional 5 minutes, or until the spinach is wilted.
- Season the soup with salt and pepper to taste.
- Ladle the soup into bowls and garnish with chopped fresh parsley before serving.

Health Benefits:

- Lentils are a good source of protein, fiber, and iron.
- Vegetables like carrots, celery, and spinach provide vitamins, minerals, and antioxidants.
- Vegetable broth is low in calories and adds flavor without added sodium.

Nutritional Value (per serving):

- Calories: 220 kcal
- Protein: 14g
- Carbohydrates: 38g
- Fat: 1g
- Fiber: 15g

Preparation Time: 40 minutes

9: Cauliflower Rice Stir-Fry

Ingredients:

- 1 medium head cauliflower
- 2 tablespoons olive oil
- 1 onion, chopped
- 2 cloves garlic, minced
- 1 bell pepper, diced
- 1 zucchini, diced
- 1 cup broccoli florets
- 1 cup sliced mushrooms
- 1/4 cup low-sodium soy sauce
- 2 tablespoons rice vinegar
- 1 tablespoon sesame oil
- 1 teaspoon grated ginger
- Salt and pepper to taste
- Sliced green onions for garnish

Instructions:

- Cut the cauliflower into florets and pulse in a food processor until it resembles rice. Set aside.

- In a large skillet or wok, heat the olive oil over medium heat. Add the chopped onion and minced garlic, and sauté until fragrant.

- Add the diced bell pepper, zucchini, broccoli florets, and sliced mushrooms to the skillet. Cook until the vegetables are tender-crisp.

- Push the vegetables to the side of the skillet and add the cauliflower rice to the center. Cook for 3-4 minutes, stirring occasionally, until the cauliflower is tender.

- In a small bowl, whisk together the low-sodium soy sauce, rice vinegar, sesame oil, and grated ginger. Pour the sauce over the stir-fry and toss to combine.

- Season with salt and pepper to taste. Garnish with sliced green onions before serving.

Health Benefits:

- Cauliflower rice is low in carbohydrates and calories, making it suitable for a renal diet.

- Colorful vegetables provide essential vitamins, minerals, and antioxidants.

- Low-sodium soy sauce adds flavor without increasing sodium intake.

Nutritional Value (per serving):

- Calories: 180 kcal

- Protein: 6g

- Carbohydrates: 14g

- Fat: 12g

- Fiber: 5g

Preparation Time: 30 minutes

10: Spinach and Chickpea Salad

Ingredients:

- 4 cups baby spinach leaves

- 1 can (15 ounces) chickpeas, rinsed and drained

- 1/2 cup cherry tomatoes, halved

- 1/4 cup red onion, thinly sliced

- 1/4 cup crumbled feta cheese

- 2 tablespoons extra virgin olive oil

- 1 tablespoon balsamic vinegar

- 1 teaspoon Dijon mustard

- Salt and pepper to taste

Instructions: In a large salad bowl, combine the baby spinach leaves, chickpeas, halved cherry tomatoes, thinly sliced red onion, and crumbled feta cheese.

- In a small bowl, whisk together the extra virgin olive oil, balsamic vinegar, Dijon mustard, salt, and pepper to make the dressing.
- Drizzle the dressing over the salad and toss gently to coat all the ingredients evenly.
- Serve immediately as a light and refreshing dinner option.

Health Benefits:

- Spinach is rich in iron, vitamins A and C, and antioxidants.
- Chickpeas provide plant-based protein and fiber, promoting satiety and aiding in digestion.
- Feta cheese adds a creamy texture and a dose of calcium.

Nutritional Value (per serving):

- Calories: 220 kcal
- Protein: 9g
- Carbohydrates: 22g
- Fat: 12g
- Fiber: 7g

Preparation Time: 15 minutes

SNACK RECIPES:

1: Cucumber Hummus Bites

Ingredients:

- 1 cucumber, sliced into rounds
- 1/2 cup hummus
- 1 tablespoon chopped fresh parsley (optional)
- Salt and pepper to taste

Instructions: Place the cucumber rounds on a serving platter.

- Spoon a small amount of hummus onto each cucumber round.
- Sprinkle chopped fresh parsley over the hummus for garnish, if desired.
- Season with salt and pepper to taste.
- Serve immediately as a refreshing and nutritious snack.

Health Benefits:

- Cucumbers are hydrating and low in potassium, making them suitable for a renal diet.
- Hummus provides plant-based protein and fiber, promoting satiety and aiding in digestion.
- Parsley adds a burst of flavor and contains vitamins A, C, and K.

Nutritional Value (per serving):

- Calories: 60 kcal
- Protein: 2g
- Carbohydrates: 7g
- Fat: 3g
- Fiber: 2g

Preparation Time: 10 minutes

2: Greek Yogurt with Berries

Ingredients:

- 1/2 cup plain Greek yogurt
- 1/4 cup mixed berries (such as strawberries, blueberries, and raspberries)
- 1 tablespoon chopped walnuts (optional)
- 1 teaspoon honey (optional)

Instructions:

- Spoon the plain Greek yogurt into a small bowl.
- Top with mixed berries and chopped walnuts.
- Drizzle with honey for added sweetness, if desired.
- Serve immediately as a protein-packed and antioxidant-rich snack.

Health Benefits:

- Greek yogurt is high in protein and calcium, supporting muscle health and bone density.
- Berries are low in potassium and high in antioxidants, protecting cells from oxidative damage.
- Walnuts provide heart-healthy omega-3 fatty acids and crunchy texture.

Nutritional Value (per serving):

- Calories: 150 kcal
- Protein: 12g
- Carbohydrates: 15g
- Fat: 6g
- Fiber: 3g

Preparation Time: 5 minutes

3: Avocado Tomato Salad

Ingredients:

- 1 ripe avocado, diced
- 1 medium tomato, diced
- 1 tablespoon chopped fresh basil
- 1 tablespoon extra virgin olive oil
- 1 teaspoon balsamic vinegar

- Salt and pepper to taste

Instructions:

- In a bowl, combine the diced avocado and tomato.
- Add chopped fresh basil, extra virgin olive oil, and balsamic vinegar.
- Season with salt and pepper to taste.
- Gently toss to coat the ingredients evenly.
- Serve immediately as a refreshing and nutrient-rich snack.

Health Benefits:

- Avocado is a source of healthy monounsaturated fats and fiber, which may help lower cholesterol levels.
- Tomatoes are rich in antioxidants, including lycopene, which may reduce the risk of chronic diseases.
- Basil adds flavor and contains essential nutrients like vitamin K and manganese.

Nutritional Value (per serving):

- Calories: 180 kcal
- Protein: 2g
- Carbohydrates: 10g
- Fat: 15g
- Fiber: 6g

Preparation Time: 10 minutes

4: Cottage Cheese with Pineapple

Ingredients:

- 1/2 cup low-fat cottage cheese
- 1/2 cup diced fresh pineapple
- 1 tablespoon chopped fresh mint (optional)
- 1 teaspoon honey (optional)
- Instructions:
- Place the low-fat cottage cheese in a bowl.
- Top with diced fresh pineapple.
- Garnish with chopped fresh mint for extra flavor, if desired.
- Drizzle with honey for sweetness, if desired.
- Serve immediately as a protein-rich and satisfying snack.

Health Benefits:

- Cottage cheese is a good source of protein and calcium, essential for muscle and bone health.
- Pineapple provides vitamin C and bromelain, an enzyme with anti-inflammatory properties.
- Mint adds a refreshing taste and may aid digestion.

Nutritional Value (per serving):

- Calories: 120 kcal

- Protein: 12g

- Carbohydrates: 15g

- Fat: 2g

- Fiber: 2g

Preparation Time: 5 minutes

5: Cucumber Hummus Bites

Ingredients:

- 1 large cucumber

- 1/2 cup hummus

- 1 tablespoon chopped fresh parsley

- Salt and pepper to taste

Instructions:

- Slice the cucumber into rounds, about 1/4-inch thick.

- Top each cucumber slice with a small dollop of hummus.

- Garnish with chopped fresh parsley.

- Season with salt and pepper to taste.

- Arrange the cucumber hummus bites on a serving platter and serve immediately.

Health Benefits:

- Cucumbers are low in calories and high in water content, providing hydration and essential vitamins.

- Hummus is a good source of plant-based protein and fiber, promoting satiety and digestive health.
- Parsley adds flavor and contains antioxidants like vitamin C and vitamin K.

Nutritional Value (per serving):

- Calories: 60 kcal
- Protein: 3g
- Carbohydrates: 8g
- Fat: 2g
- Fiber: 2g

Preparation Time: 10 minutes

6: Greek Yogurt Berry Parfait

Ingredients:

- 1/2 cup plain Greek yogurt
- 1/4 cup mixed berries (such as strawberries, blueberries, raspberries)
- 1 tablespoon chopped nuts (such as almonds, walnuts)
- 1 teaspoon honey (optional)

Instructions:

- In a glass or bowl, layer the plain Greek yogurt.
- Top with mixed berries.

- Sprinkle chopped nuts over the berries.
- Drizzle with honey for added sweetness, if desired.
- Repeat the layers if desired, ending with a sprinkle of nuts on top.
- Serve immediately as a nutritious and satisfying snack.

Health Benefits:

- Greek yogurt is rich in protein and probiotics, promoting gut health and providing essential nutrients.
- Berries are packed with antioxidants, fiber, and vitamins, supporting heart health and immune function.
- Nuts are a good source of healthy fats, protein, and micronutrients, contributing to satiety and overall health.

Nutritional Value (per serving):

- Calories: 150 kcal
- Protein: 10g
- Carbohydrates: 15g
- Fat: 6g
- Fiber: 3g

Preparation Time: 5 minutes

7: Avocado Tomato Salad

Ingredients:

- 1 ripe avocado, diced

- 1 medium tomato, diced

- 1/4 cup diced cucumber

- 2 tablespoons chopped fresh cilantro

- 1 tablespoon lemon juice

- Salt and pepper to taste

Instructions:

- In a mixing bowl, combine the diced avocado, tomato, cucumber, and chopped cilantro.

- Drizzle lemon juice over the mixture and gently toss to combine.

- Season with salt and pepper to taste.

- Serve immediately as a refreshing and nutritious snack option.

Health Benefits:

- Avocado is rich in heart-healthy monounsaturated fats, fiber, and potassium, supporting overall health and kidney function.

- Tomatoes are high in antioxidants like lycopene, which may help reduce inflammation and lower the risk of chronic diseases.

- Cucumber adds hydration and essential vitamins and minerals, contributing to overall well-being.

Nutritional Value (per serving):

- Calories: 120 kcal

- Protein: 2g

- Carbohydrates: 8g

- Fat: 10g

- Fiber: 5g

Preparation Time: 10 minutes

8: Mediterranean Veggie Skewers

Ingredients:

- 1 small zucchini, sliced into rounds

- 1 bell pepper, cut into chunks

- 1 cup cherry tomatoes

- 1/2 red onion, cut into chunks

- 2 tablespoons olive oil

- 1 teaspoon dried oregano

- Salt and pepper to taste

Instructions:

- Preheat the grill or grill pan over medium heat.
- Thread the zucchini rounds, bell pepper chunks, cherry tomatoes, and red onion chunks onto skewers.
- Brush the vegetable skewers with olive oil and sprinkle with dried oregano, salt, and pepper.
- Grill the skewers for 8-10 minutes, turning occasionally, until the vegetables are tender and lightly charred.
- Remove from the grill and serve immediately as a flavorful and nutritious snack.

Health Benefits:

- Zucchini is low in calories and rich in vitamins A and C, promoting eye health and immune function.
- Bell peppers are packed with vitamin C, antioxidants, and fiber, supporting heart health and digestion.
- Cherry tomatoes are high in lycopene and vitamin K, providing anti-inflammatory and bone-strengthening benefits.

Nutritional Value (per serving):

- Calories: 80 kcal
- Protein: 2g
- Carbohydrates: 8g

- Fat: 5g
- Fiber: 3g

Preparation Time: 15 minutes

9: Greek Yogurt Berry Parfait

Ingredients:

- 1/2 cup low-fat Greek yogurt
- 1/4 cup mixed berries (such as strawberries, blueberries, and raspberries)
- 2 tablespoons chopped nuts (such as almonds or walnuts)
- 1 teaspoon honey or maple syrup (optional)
- 1/2 teaspoon vanilla extract

Instructions:

- In a small bowl or glass, layer the Greek yogurt, mixed berries, and chopped nuts.
- Drizzle with honey or maple syrup if desired and sprinkle with vanilla extract.
- Repeat the layers until all ingredients are used.
- Serve immediately as a refreshing and protein-packed snack.
- Health Benefits:
- Greek yogurt is high in protein and calcium, supporting bone health and muscle function.

- Berries are rich in antioxidants and fiber, helping to reduce inflammation and improve digestive health.

- Nuts provide healthy fats and essential nutrients, promoting heart health and satiety.

- Nutritional Value (per serving):

- Calories: 180 kcal

- Protein: 12g

- Carbohydrates: 15g

- Fat: 8g

- Fiber: 3g

Preparation Time: 5 minutes

10: Cucumber Hummus Bites

Ingredients:

- 1 English cucumber, sliced into rounds

- 1/2 cup hummus (store-bought or homemade)

- 2 tablespoons chopped fresh parsley or dill

- Pinch of paprika or cumin for garnish (optional)

Instructions:

- Place the cucumber rounds on a serving platter.

- Spoon a dollop of hummus onto each cucumber round.

- Sprinkle with chopped parsley or dill and garnish with a pinch of paprika or cumin if desired.
- Serve immediately as a crunchy and satisfying snack option.

Health Benefits: Cucumber is low in calories and high in water content, aiding hydration and providing essential vitamins and minerals.

- Hummus is a good source of plant-based protein and fiber, helping to regulate blood sugar levels and support digestive health.
- Fresh herbs like parsley and dill add flavor and nutrients, including vitamins A and K.

Nutritional Value (per serving):

- Calories: 70 kcal
- Protein: 3g
- Carbohydrates: 9g
- Fat: 3g
- Fiber: 2g

Preparation Time: 10 minutes

1: Baked Apples with Cinnamon

Ingredients:

- 2 medium-sized apples
- 1 tablespoon unsalted butter or coconut oil, melted
- 1 teaspoon ground cinnamon
- 1 tablespoon chopped walnuts or almonds (optional)
- 1 tablespoon honey or maple syrup (optional)

Instructions:

- Preheat the oven to 375°F (190°C).
- Core the apples and remove the seeds, leaving the bottoms intact.
- In a small bowl, mix the melted butter or coconut oil with cinnamon.
- Place the cored apples in a baking dish and brush them with the cinnamon mixture, ensuring they are evenly coated.
- If desired, sprinkle chopped nuts over the top of each apple and drizzle with honey or maple syrup.
- Bake for 25-30 minutes, or until the apples are tender and lightly browned.
- Serve warm and enjoy this comforting and naturally sweet dessert.

Health Benefits:

- Apples are rich in fiber and antioxidants, supporting digestive health and reducing inflammation.
- Cinnamon helps regulate blood sugar levels and may improve insulin sensitivity.
- Nuts provide healthy fats and protein, promoting heart health and satiety.

Nutritional Value (per serving):

- Calories: 150 kcal
- Protein: 1g
- Carbohydrates: 30g
- Fat: 5g
- Fiber: 5g

Preparation Time: 35 minutes

2: Berry Chia Seed Pudding

Ingredients:

- 1/4 cup chia seeds
- 1 cup unsweetened almond milk or coconut milk
- 1/2 teaspoon vanilla extract
- 1 tablespoon honey or maple syrup (optional)

- 1/2 cup mixed berries (such as strawberries, blueberries, and raspberries)

Instructions:

- In a mixing bowl, combine the chia seeds, almond milk, vanilla extract, and sweetener (if using). Stir well to combine.
- Cover the bowl and refrigerate for at least 2 hours, or preferably overnight, to allow the chia seeds to absorb the liquid and thicken.
- Once the pudding has reached the desired consistency, remove it from the refrigerator and give it a good stir.
- Spoon the pudding into serving bowls or glasses and top with mixed berries.
- Serve chilled and enjoy this refreshing and nutritious dessert option.

Health Benefits:

- Chia seeds are high in fiber and omega-3 fatty acids, promoting digestive health and reducing inflammation.
- Berries are packed with antioxidants and vitamins, supporting immune function and overall well-being.

- Almond milk or coconut milk are low in calories and dairy-free, making them suitable options for those with lactose intolerance or dairy sensitivities.

Nutritional Value (per serving):

- Calories: 150 kcal

- Protein: 4g

- Carbohydrates: 20g

- Fat: 7g

- Fiber: 10g

Preparation Time: 2 hours (including chilling time)

3: Baked Apples with Cinnamon and Walnuts

Ingredients:

- 2 medium apples (such as Granny Smith or Fuji)

- 2 tablespoons chopped walnuts

- 1 tablespoon honey or maple syrup (optional)

- 1/2 teaspoon ground cinnamon

- 1/4 teaspoon nutmeg

- 1 teaspoon lemon juice

- 1 teaspoon unsalted butter or coconut oil

Instructions: Preheat the oven to 375°F (190°C). Core the apples, leaving the bottoms intact.

- In a small bowl, mix the chopped walnuts, honey or maple syrup (if using), ground cinnamon, and nutmeg.
- Stuff the center of each apple with the walnut mixture.
- Drizzle lemon juice over the stuffed apples and dot with butter or coconut oil.
- Place the apples in a baking dish and bake for 25-30 minutes or until tender.
- Serve warm, optionally topped with a dollop of Greek yogurt or a sprinkle of additional cinnamon.

Health Benefits:

- Apples are rich in fiber and antioxidants, supporting digestive health and reducing inflammation.
- Walnuts provide omega-3 fatty acids and vitamin E, promoting heart health and cognitive function.
- Cinnamon may help regulate blood sugar levels and improve insulin sensitivity.

Nutritional Value (per serving, without optional toppings):

- Calories: 150 kcal
- Protein: 2g
- Carbohydrates: 26g
- Fat: 6g
- Fiber: 5g

Preparation Time: 40 minutes

4: Chia Seed Pudding with Berries

Ingredients:

- 2 tablespoons chia seeds
- 1/2 cup unsweetened almond milk or coconut milk
- 1/4 teaspoon vanilla extract
- 1 teaspoon honey or maple syrup (optional)
- 1/2 cup mixed berries (such as strawberries, blueberries, and raspberries)
- Fresh mint leaves for garnish (optional)

Instructions:

- In a bowl, mix the chia seeds, almond milk or coconut milk, vanilla extract, and honey or maple syrup (if using). Stir well to combine.
- Let the mixture sit for 5 minutes, then stir again to prevent clumping. Refrigerate for at least 2 hours or overnight to thicken.
- Once the chia pudding has set, divide it into serving bowls or glasses.
- Top each serving with mixed berries and garnish with fresh mint leaves if desired.
- Serve chilled as a refreshing and nutritious dessert option.

Health Benefits:

- Chia seeds are packed with fiber, protein, and omega-3 fatty acids, supporting digestive health and reducing inflammation.

- Berries are rich in antioxidants and vitamins, promoting heart health and cognitive function.

- Almond milk or coconut milk provide calcium and vitamin D, supporting bone health.

Nutritional Value (per serving):

- Calories: 120 kcal

- Protein: 3g

- Carbohydrates: 14g

- Fat: 6g

- Fiber: 8g

Preparation Time: 5 minutes (plus chilling time)

5: Baked Pears with Almonds and Honey

Ingredients:

- 2 ripe but firm pears

- 2 tablespoons sliced almonds

- 1 tablespoon honey

- 1/2 teaspoon ground cinnamon

- 1/4 teaspoon ground ginger

- 1 teaspoon lemon juice

- 1 teaspoon unsalted butter or coconut oil

Instructions:

- Preheat the oven to 375°F (190°C). Cut the pears in half lengthwise and remove the cores.

- Place the pear halves cut side up in a baking dish. Drizzle lemon juice over the pears.

- In a small bowl, mix together the sliced almonds, honey, ground cinnamon, and ground ginger.

- Spoon the almond mixture into the center of each pear half. Dot with butter or coconut oil.

- Bake for 20-25 minutes, or until the pears are tender and the topping is golden brown.

- Serve warm, optionally topped with a dollop of Greek yogurt or a sprinkle of additional cinnamon.

Health Benefits:

- Pears are rich in fiber and vitamin C, supporting digestive health and boosting immunity.

- Almonds provide healthy fats, protein, and vitamin E, promoting heart health and satiety.

- Cinnamon and ginger offer anti-inflammatory properties and may help regulate blood sugar levels.

Nutritional Value (per serving, without optional toppings):

- Calories: 150 kcal
- Protein: 3g
- Carbohydrates: 25g
- Fat: 6g
- Fiber: 6g

Preparation Time: 30 minutes

6: Greek Yogurt Parfait with Berries and Almonds

Ingredients:

- 1/2 cup plain Greek yogurt
- 1/4 cup mixed berries (such as strawberries, blueberries, and raspberries)
- 2 tablespoons sliced almonds
- 1 tablespoon honey or maple syrup (optional)
- 1/4 teaspoon vanilla extract

Instructions:

- In a serving glass or bowl, layer the Greek yogurt, mixed berries, and sliced almonds.

- Drizzle honey or maple syrup (if using) over the layers and sprinkle with vanilla extract.
- Repeat the layering process until all ingredients are used, ending with a sprinkle of sliced almonds on top.
- Serve immediately as a nutritious and satisfying dessert option.

Health Benefits: Greek yogurt is high in protein and probiotics, supporting gut health and providing essential nutrients.

- Berries are packed with antioxidants and fiber, promoting heart health and reducing inflammation.
- Almonds offer healthy fats, protein, and vitamin E, supporting brain function and satiety.

Nutritional Value (per serving):

- Calories: 180 kcal
- Protein: 12g
- Carbohydrates: 15g
- Fat: 8g
- Fiber: 4g

Preparation Time: 5 minutes

7: Chia Seed Pudding with Coconut and Mango

Ingredients:

- 2 tablespoons chia seeds
- 1/2 cup unsweetened almond milk
- 1/4 teaspoon vanilla extract
- 1/4 cup diced mango
- 1 tablespoon shredded coconut
- 1 teaspoon honey or maple syrup (optional)

Instructions: In a small bowl or jar, mix together the chia seeds, almond milk, and vanilla extract. Let it sit for 5 minutes.

- Stir the mixture again to prevent clumping, then cover and refrigerate overnight or for at least 2 hours until thickened.
- Once the chia pudding has set, layer it in serving glasses or bowls with diced mango and shredded coconut.
- Drizzle with honey or maple syrup (if using) for added sweetness.
- Serve chilled as a refreshing and nutrient-rich dessert option.

Health Benefits:

- Chia seeds are rich in fiber and omega-3 fatty acids, supporting digestive health and reducing inflammation.
- Mangoes are high in vitamin C and antioxidants, promoting immune function and skin health.

- Coconut provides healthy fats and medium-chain triglycerides (MCTs), which can support brain health and metabolism.

Nutritional Value (per serving):

- Calories: 180 kcal
- Protein: 4g
- Carbohydrates: 22g
- Fat: 8g
- Fiber: 9g

Preparation Time: 5 minutes (plus chilling time)

8: Avocado Chocolate Mousse

Ingredients:

- 1 ripe avocado
- 2 tablespoons unsweetened cocoa powder
- 2 tablespoons honey or maple syrup
- 1/4 teaspoon vanilla extract
- Pinch of salt
- Fresh berries, for garnish (optional)

Instructions:

- Cut the avocado in half, remove the pit, and scoop the flesh into a blender or food processor.

- Add the cocoa powder, honey or maple syrup, vanilla extract, and a pinch of salt to the blender.

- Blend until smooth and creamy, scraping down the sides of the blender as needed.

- Transfer the chocolate mousse to serving bowls or glasses.

- Refrigerate for at least 30 minutes to chill and set.

- Garnish with fresh berries before serving, if desired.

Health Benefits:

- Avocados are rich in heart-healthy monounsaturated fats and potassium, supporting cardiovascular health and blood pressure regulation.

- Cocoa powder is high in antioxidants and flavonoids, which have been linked to improved heart health and cognitive function.

Nutritional Value (per serving, without optional toppings):

- Calories: 180 kcal

- Protein: 3g

- Carbohydrates: 19g

- Fat: 12g

- Fiber: 7g

Preparation Time: 10 minutes

9: Berry Yogurt Parfait

Ingredients:

- 1/2 cup low-fat plain Greek yogurt
- 1/4 cup mixed berries (such as strawberries, blueberries, and raspberries)
- 2 tablespoons chopped nuts (such as almonds or walnuts)
- 1 tablespoon unsweetened shredded coconut
- 1 teaspoon honey or maple syrup (optional)

Instructions:

- In a serving glass or bowl, layer the Greek yogurt, mixed berries, chopped nuts, and shredded coconut.
- Repeat the layers until all ingredients are used, ending with a sprinkle of shredded coconut on top.
- Drizzle with honey or maple syrup (if using) for added sweetness.
- Serve immediately as a refreshing and nutrient-rich dessert option.

Health Benefits:

- Greek yogurt provides protein and probiotics, supporting digestive health and muscle maintenance.
- Berries are rich in antioxidants and vitamins, promoting immune function and reducing inflammation.

- Nuts offer healthy fats and fiber, aiding in heart health and satiety.

Nutritional Value (per serving):

- Calories: 180 kcal
- Protein: 12g
- Carbohydrates: 15g
- Fat: 8g
- Fiber: 4g

Preparation Time: 5 minutes

10: Baked Apples with Cinnamon and Almonds

Ingredients:

- 2 medium-sized apples, cored and halved
- 1 tablespoon lemon juice
- 1/2 teaspoon ground cinnamon
- 2 tablespoons chopped almonds
- 1 teaspoon honey or maple syrup (optional)

Instructions:

- Preheat the oven to 375°F (190°C). Line a baking dish with parchment paper or lightly coat with cooking spray.
- Place the apple halves in the prepared baking dish and drizzle with lemon juice to prevent browning.

- Sprinkle ground cinnamon evenly over the apple halves, then top with chopped almonds.
- Drizzle with honey or maple syrup (if using) for added sweetness.
- Bake in the preheated oven for 20-25 minutes, or until the apples are tender and lightly browned.
- Remove from the oven and let cool slightly before serving.
- Serve warm as a comforting and nutritious dessert option.

Health Benefits: Apples are a good source of fiber and vitamin C, promoting digestive health and immune function.

- Cinnamon may help regulate blood sugar levels and improve insulin sensitivity.
- Almonds provide healthy fats and protein, supporting heart health and satiety.

Nutritional Value (per serving):

- Calories: 150 kcal
- Protein: 3g
- Carbohydrates: 20g
- Fat: 7g
- Fiber: 5g

Preparation Time: 30 minutes

CHAPTER THREE: Nutrition and CKD

Basics of Renal Diet

The basics of a renal diet are tailored to support kidney health and manage the symptoms associated with chronic kidney disease (CKD), particularly in Stage 4. Here are key principles of a renal diet:

Sodium Restriction: Limiting sodium intake is crucial for individuals with CKD as it helps control blood pressure and reduce fluid retention. A renal diet typically involves avoiding processed and high-sodium foods, such as canned soups, processed meats, and salty snacks.

Protein Moderation: Consuming an appropriate amount of high-quality protein is important for maintaining muscle mass and overall health. However, individuals with CKD may need to moderate their protein intake, as excessive protein consumption can strain the kidneys. A renal diet typically includes lean protein sources such as poultry, fish, and tofu, and limits intake of red meats and dairy products.

Phosphorus Control: In advanced stages of CKD, impaired kidney function can lead to elevated phosphorus levels in the blood, which can contribute to bone and cardiovascular complications.

A renal diet focuses on limiting phosphorus-rich foods such as dairy products, nuts, and processed foods containing phosphate additives.

Potassium Management: Abnormal potassium levels are common in CKD, with high levels posing a risk of cardiac arrhythmias and low levels leading to muscle weakness. A renal diet aims to regulate potassium intake by limiting potassium-rich foods such as bananas, oranges, potatoes, and tomatoes.

Fluid Restriction: Individuals with CKD may need to limit fluid intake to prevent fluid overload and swelling. This typically involves monitoring fluid intake from beverages and foods with high water content, such as soups, fruits, and vegetables.

Individualized Approach: A renal diet should be tailored to the individual's specific nutritional needs, medical history, stage of CKD, and treatment plan. Working closely with a registered dietitian or healthcare provider is essential to develop a personalized renal diet plan that meets the individual's dietary requirements while supporting kidney health.

By following the basics of a renal diet, individuals with Stage 4 CKD can help manage their condition, reduce symptoms, and improve overall quality of life.

Nutritional Needs for Stage 4 CKD

In Stage 4 chronic kidney disease (CKD), the kidneys have significantly reduced function, and individuals may experience various nutritional challenges.

Meeting specific nutritional needs becomes essential to manage symptoms, slow disease progression, and improve overall health. Here are key considerations for the nutritional needs of individuals with Stage 4 CKD:

Protein: While protein is essential for maintaining muscle mass and supporting overall health, individuals with Stage 4 CKD may need to moderate their protein intake. High protein consumption can increase the burden on the kidneys and exacerbate symptoms. However, adequate protein intake is still necessary. Thus, it's crucial to work with a dietitian to determine the appropriate amount and source of protein based on individual needs.

Sodium: Sodium restriction is crucial for managing blood pressure and fluid balance in individuals with CKD. Excessive sodium intake can lead to fluid retention and worsen hypertension. Therefore, limiting sodium-rich foods such as processed and packaged foods, canned soups, and salty snacks is essential.

Phosphorus and Potassium: Abnormal levels of phosphorus and potassium are common in Stage 4 CKD.

Elevated phosphorus levels can contribute to bone and cardiovascular complications, while imbalanced potassium levels can affect heart function. Therefore, it's important to moderate the intake of phosphorus-rich foods like dairy products and limit high-potassium foods such as bananas, potatoes, and tomatoes.

Fluids: Fluid intake may need to be restricted in individuals with Stage 4 CKD to prevent fluid overload and manage symptoms like swelling and high blood pressure. Monitoring fluid intake from both beverages and foods with high water content is essential.

Individualized Approach: Nutritional needs can vary depending on factors such as age, gender, weight, medical history, and treatment plan. Therefore, a personalized approach to nutrition, tailored to the individual's specific needs and preferences, is crucial. Working closely with a registered dietitian or healthcare provider can help develop a customized nutrition plan that supports kidney health and overall well-being.

Importance of Portion Control

Portion control plays a crucial role in managing Stage 4 chronic kidney disease (CKD) by helping individuals maintain a balanced diet, control symptoms, and slow disease progression. Here's why portion control is important for individuals with Stage 4 CKD:

Managing Nutrient Intake: Controlling portion sizes ensures that individuals consume appropriate amounts of essential nutrients while avoiding excessive intake of nutrients that may be harmful. With CKD, moderation is key, as overconsumption of certain nutrients like protein, sodium, phosphorus, and potassium can exacerbate symptoms and contribute to complications.

Controlling Caloric Intake: Portion control helps regulate calorie intake, which is important for managing weight and preventing obesity-related complications such as diabetes and cardiovascular disease. Excess weight can strain the kidneys and worsen CKD symptoms, so maintaining a healthy weight through portion control is essential.

Preventing Fluid Overload: For individuals with CKD, fluid restriction may be necessary to manage symptoms like edema (swelling) and high blood pressure. Monitoring portion sizes of fluid-rich foods like soups, fruits, and vegetables can help prevent fluid overload and maintain fluid balance in the body.

Supporting Blood Sugar Control: Controlling portion sizes of carbohydrate-rich foods is important for managing blood sugar levels, especially for individuals with diabetes, which is a common complication of CKD. Consistent carbohydrate intake throughout the day helps prevent blood sugar spikes and promotes better glucose control.

Improving Digestive Health: Eating large portions can put stress on the digestive system, leading to discomfort, bloating, and other gastrointestinal issues.

Portion control promotes better digestion and absorption of nutrients, reducing the risk of digestive problems commonly experienced by individuals with CKD.

Overall, practicing portion control empowers individuals with Stage 4 CKD to make informed dietary choices, optimize nutrient intake, and effectively manage their condition to improve quality of life and long-term health outcomes.

CHAPTER FOUR: Meal Planning Tips

Guidelines for Meal Planning

Meal planning is a crucial aspect of managing Stage 4 CKD, as it helps individuals maintain a balanced diet while adhering to dietary restrictions necessary for kidney health. Here are some guidelines to consider when planning meals for seniors with Stage 4 CKD:

Monitor Nutrient Intake: Ensure that meals are nutritionally balanced, focusing on controlling protein, sodium, potassium, and phosphorus levels. Aim for adequate protein intake while limiting high-potassium and high-phosphorus foods.

Portion Control: Practice portion control to prevent overconsumption of nutrients that may be harmful to kidney function. Use measuring tools and guidelines to portion out appropriate servings of proteins, grains, fruits, and vegetables.

Choose Low-Potassium Foods: Opt for low-potassium foods such as apples, berries, green beans, and cabbage. Limit high-potassium foods like bananas, oranges, tomatoes, and potatoes, as excess potassium can be harmful to individuals with compromised kidney function.

Limit Phosphorus Intake: Select foods that are lower in phosphorus to prevent the buildup of phosphorus in the blood. Foods such as white bread, rice, pasta, and certain fruits and vegetables are lower in phosphorus compared to dairy products, nuts, seeds, and processed foods.

Reduce Sodium: Minimize sodium intake by using herbs, spices, and lemon juice to flavor meals instead of salt. Avoid processed and packaged foods, which are typically high in sodium, and opt for fresh, whole ingredients whenever possible.

Include a Variety of Foods: Incorporate a diverse range of foods to ensure adequate nutrient intake and prevent monotony in meals. Rotate through different grains, proteins, fruits, and vegetables to provide variety and flavor.

Stay Hydrated: Encourage adequate fluid intake, but monitor fluid intake closely, as excessive fluid consumption can strain the kidneys. Offer hydrating options such as water, herbal teas, and diluted fruit juices throughout the day.

By following these guidelines for meal planning, individuals with Stage 4 CKD can support kidney health while enjoying delicious and nutritious meals tailored to their dietary needs.

Creating Balanced Meals

Creating balanced meals for individuals with Stage 4 CKD involves careful consideration of nutrient content and portion sizes to support kidney health while providing essential nutrients. Here are some key principles to keep in mind when designing balanced meals:

Focus on High-Quality Protein: Choose lean sources of protein such as poultry, fish, eggs, and plant-based sources like tofu and legumes. These provide essential amino acids without excessive phosphorus and potassium, which can be harmful in high amounts for individuals with compromised kidney function.

Include Low-Potassium Foods: Select fruits and vegetables that are lower in potassium to avoid potassium buildup in the bloodstream. Examples include apples, berries, cucumbers, and green beans. Limit high-potassium options like bananas, oranges, tomatoes, and potatoes.

Manage Phosphorus Intake: Be mindful of phosphorus content, as excessive phosphorus can contribute to bone and heart health issues. Choose dairy alternatives like almond milk, limit intake of high-phosphorus foods such as cheese and processed meats, and opt for whole grains over refined grains.

Control Sodium Levels: Reduce sodium intake to support heart and kidney health by cooking from scratch using fresh ingredients and avoiding processed and canned foods, which are often high in sodium. Use herbs, spices, and lemon juice to add flavor without salt.

Incorporate Whole Grains: Choose whole grains like brown rice, quinoa, and whole wheat bread over refined grains to provide fiber and essential nutrients while keeping phosphorus levels in check.

Balance Plate Composition: Aim for a balanced plate composition with half filled with non-starchy vegetables, a quarter with protein, and a quarter with whole grains or starchy vegetables. This helps control portion sizes and ensures a variety of nutrients.

Monitor Fluid Intake: Encourage adequate but controlled fluid intake to prevent dehydration and fluid overload. Offer fluids throughout the day and limit intake during meals to avoid overwhelming the kidneys.

By following these principles, individuals with Stage 4 CKD can enjoy balanced meals that support overall health and kidney function. Consulting with a healthcare provider or dietitian can provide personalized guidance based on individual needs and medical history.

Tips for Eating Out

Eating out can present challenges for individuals with Stage 4 CKD, as restaurant meals often contain high amounts of sodium, phosphorus, and potassium, which can be harmful for kidney health. However, with some planning and mindfulness, it's still possible to enjoy dining out while adhering to dietary restrictions. Here are some tips for eating out with Stage 4 CKD:

Research Restaurants: Prior to dining out, research restaurants in advance to find ones that offer options suitable for a renal diet.

Look for restaurants that prioritize fresh ingredients and offer customizable dishes.

Choose Wisely: Opt for restaurants that offer a variety of dishes with simple, whole-food ingredients. Select items that are grilled, baked, or steamed rather than fried or heavily processed. Look for menu items labeled as low-sodium or renal-friendly.

Ask Questions: Don't hesitate to ask your server about menu ingredients and preparation methods. Inquire about options for substitutions or modifications to accommodate your dietary needs. Most restaurants are willing to accommodate special requests.

Control Portions: Restaurant portions are often oversized, so consider sharing an entree with a dining companion or requesting a half portion. This helps control portion sizes and reduces the intake of potentially harmful nutrients.

Limit Sodium: Request that your meal be prepared with minimal added salt, and ask for sauces, dressings, and condiments on the side so you can control the amount added. Avoid dishes that are typically high in sodium, such as soups, cured meats, and heavily seasoned dishes.

Be Mindful of Condiments: Be cautious with condiments like soy sauce, ketchup, and barbecue sauce, as they can be high in sodium and phosphorus. Use them sparingly or ask for low-sodium alternatives.

Stay Hydrated: Be mindful of your fluid intake, especially if you're dining at a restaurant that serves alcoholic beverages or salty foods. Drink water or other kidney-friendly beverages to stay hydrated without overloading on fluids.

By following these tips, individuals with Stage 4 CKD can navigate restaurant menus with confidence and enjoy dining out without compromising their renal diet.

Cooking Techniques for Renal Diet

When it comes to cooking for individuals with Stage 4 CKD, it's essential to adopt specific techniques that support their dietary restrictions and nutritional needs. Here are some cooking techniques tailored for a renal diet:

Limiting Salt: Excessive sodium intake can exacerbate hypertension and fluid retention, common concerns for CKD patients. To reduce salt in recipes, use herbs, spices, and citrus juices to add flavor instead. Fresh herbs like basil, parsley, and cilantro can enhance the taste of dishes without relying on salt.

Boiling and Steaming: Boiling and steaming are preferred methods for cooking vegetables, grains, and proteins in a renal diet. These techniques help retain nutrients while minimizing the need for added fats or oils. Vegetables like carrots, broccoli, and cauliflower can be steamed to preserve their texture and flavor.

Trimming Fat: High-fat meats and dairy products can contribute to cardiovascular issues, which are often comorbidities with CKD. Opt for lean cuts of meat, remove visible fat, and choose low-fat or fat-free dairy options when cooking. Grilling, broiling, or baking meats can render out excess fat while still providing a satisfying flavor.

Monitoring Phosphorus: Phosphorus is another nutrient that needs careful attention in renal diets. To reduce phosphorus content in meals, consider soaking beans and legumes before cooking, as this can help leach out some of the phosphorus. Additionally, choosing fresh fruits and vegetables over processed or canned varieties can help minimize phosphorus intake.

Limiting Potassium: Potassium levels should also be monitored in CKD patients, especially in later stages. To reduce potassium in recipes, opt for cooking methods that leach out potassium, such as boiling potatoes or vegetables and discarding the cooking water. Also, incorporating low-potassium alternatives like apples, berries, and green beans can help balance potassium intake.

Portion Control: Controlling portion sizes is crucial in managing nutrient intake for CKD patients. Use measuring cups, spoons, and kitchen scales to portion out ingredients accurately, and consider serving meals on smaller plates to encourage mindful eating.

By employing these cooking techniques, individuals with Stage 4 CKD can enjoy flavorful and nutritious meals while adhering to their dietary restrictions and promoting overall health and well-being.

Ingredient Substitutions

In a renal diet tailored for individuals with Stage 4 CKD, ingredient substitutions play a vital role in managing nutrient intake and supporting overall health. Here are some common ingredient substitutions to consider:

Salt Substitutes: Instead of using table salt, which is high in sodium, opt for salt substitutes that are potassium-based. These substitutes mimic the taste of salt without contributing to sodium levels. However, it's essential to consult with a healthcare provider before using salt substitutes, especially for individuals with potassium restrictions.

Herbs and Spices: Herbs and spices are excellent alternatives to salt for adding flavor to dishes. Fresh herbs like basil, parsley, cilantro, and dill can enhance the taste of meals without increasing sodium intake. Spices such as cinnamon, cumin, turmeric, and ginger can also add depth and complexity to recipes.

Low-Sodium Broth: Instead of using regular broth or stock, opt for low-sodium varieties when preparing soups, stews, and sauces.

Alternatively, you can make homemade broth using fresh vegetables and herbs to control sodium levels.

Whole Grains: Whole grains are a valuable source of fiber and nutrients, but some varieties may be high in phosphorus and potassium.

Consider substituting high-phosphorus grains like brown rice with lower-phosphorus options such as white rice or bulgur. Quinoa and barley are also good alternatives that provide nutritional benefits without excess phosphorus or potassium.

Low-Potassium Fruits and Vegetables: While fruits and vegetables are essential components of a healthy diet, some varieties are high in potassium, which may need to be limited for individuals with CKD.

Opt for low-potassium options like apples, berries, grapes, cauliflower, and green beans. Additionally, cooking methods such as boiling or soaking can help reduce potassium levels in certain vegetables.

Lean Protein Sources: For individuals with CKD, it's essential to choose lean protein sources to reduce phosphorus and fat intake. Substitute high-fat meats with lean cuts of poultry, fish, or tofu. Legumes, such as beans and lentils, are also excellent plant-based protein alternatives that are low in phosphorus and saturated fat.

By making thoughtful ingredient substitutions, individuals with Stage 4 CKD can enjoy flavorful and nutritious meals while adhering to their dietary restrictions and supporting their overall health and well-being.

Hydration and CKD

Hydration plays a crucial role in managing chronic kidney disease (CKD), especially for individuals in Stage 4 CKD. Proper hydration is essential for maintaining kidney function, preventing complications, and promoting overall health and well-being.

In Stage 4 CKD, the kidneys are significantly impaired, leading to a reduced ability to regulate fluid balance in the body. As a result, individuals with CKD are at higher risk of dehydration, electrolyte imbalances, and other complications related to inadequate fluid intake.

Maintaining optimal hydration levels is vital for several reasons. Firstly, adequate hydration helps to support kidney function by ensuring a steady flow of blood to the kidneys, which is necessary for filtering waste products and excess fluids from the bloodstream. Proper hydration also helps to prevent the formation of kidney stones, a common complication of CKD.

Furthermore, staying well-hydrated can help alleviate symptoms associated with CKD, such as fatigue, muscle cramps, and dizziness. It can also improve overall energy levels and cognitive function.

However, individuals with Stage 4 CKD need to be mindful of their fluid intake, as consuming too much fluid can put added strain on the kidneys and worsen fluid retention and swelling.

Therefore, it's essential for individuals with CKD to strike a balance between staying adequately hydrated and avoiding excessive fluid intake.

To maintain proper hydration levels, individuals with Stage 4 CKD should aim to drink enough fluids throughout the day, but the amount should be tailored to their specific needs and recommendations provided by their healthcare provider or dietitian. In some cases, fluid intake may need to be restricted, especially if there are concerns about fluid retention or electrolyte imbalances.

Choosing hydrating beverages such as water, herbal teas, and diluted fruit juices can help meet fluid needs without adding unnecessary calories or sugars.

Additionally, monitoring urine output and paying attention to signs of dehydration or overhydration can help individuals with CKD maintain optimal hydration levels and support kidney health.

CONCLUSION

The Stage 4 Renal Diet Cookbook for Seniors serves as a valuable resource for individuals navigating the complexities of chronic kidney disease (CKD) in its advanced stages.

Through a carefully curated collection of nutritious and delicious recipes, this cookbook empowers seniors with CKD to take control of their health and well-being by making informed dietary choices.

By focusing on low-potassium, low-phosphorus, and low-sodium ingredients, these recipes are tailored to meet the unique nutritional needs of individuals with Stage 4 CKD, helping to alleviate symptoms, manage complications, and slow the progression of the disease.

Each recipe is thoughtfully crafted to provide essential nutrients while limiting substances that may exacerbate kidney function decline.

Furthermore, this cookbook emphasizes the importance of portion control, hydration management, and mindful eating habits, offering practical tips and guidance to support individuals with CKD in making sustainable lifestyle changes. Whether it's a nourishing breakfast to start the day, a satisfying lunch to fuel the afternoon, or a comforting dinner to unwind in the evening, these recipes are designed to nourish the body and soothe the soul.

Beyond its culinary offerings, this cookbook also serves as a comprehensive guide to understanding CKD, providing essential information on managing symptoms, monitoring kidney function, and adopting healthy lifestyle habits.

With its wealth of knowledge and practical advice, it empowers seniors with CKD to take charge of their health and embrace a fulfilling and vibrant life, despite the challenges posed by their condition.

In essence, the Stage 4 Renal Diet Cookbook for Seniors is more than just a collection of recipes—it's a roadmap to better health and well-being, offering hope, support, and inspiration to individuals on their journey towards kidney health and vitality.

Whether you're a senior with CKD, a caregiver, or a healthcare professional, this cookbook is an indispensable resource for promoting kidney health and enhancing quality of life.